Essential Oils for Women Over 50

35 Recipes for Any Situation

Table of Contents

Introduction

You get out of bed in the morning, and you feel some aches run through your body. You reach for your toothbrush and as you brush your teeth, you notice that both your hand and wrist ache, and your face is getting wrinkly.

You bend over to put on your shoes, and you feel the aches in every joint of your body.

You don't know what happened. It seems that it was only yesterday that you were young – enjoying all the wild things life had to offer without giving a thought to your age or your body.

But now, now that you have passed 50 you feel things beginning to change. There are aches and pains where there weren't any before. You feel tired and winded when you didn't before. You still love your life, but there is a different tone that you didn't feel before.

What is happening?

While you can't stop getting older, you can stop the effects getting older has on your body. You don't have to age in your body like you are aging in your mind, and you don't have to live life with aches and pains.

If you take the right care of your body, you can naturally ward off all the aches and pains that you feel, and you can do it without stress, without chemicals, and without spending a lot of money on treatments that don't work any better than the natural way anyway.

With essential oils, you are going to learn exactly what you need to do to feel and look younger, and to embrace that youthful glow you once had. You might not be able to stop getting older, but with these blends, you are going to feel younger, happier, and healthier while you save money.

There's nothing more valuable than your health, and with these essential oils, you're going to recover your health like never before.

Let's get started.

Chapter 1 – The Oil Blends

Blend of Youth

What you will need:

10 drops frankincense

12 drops rose oil

Directions:

In a small jar, combine all oils and shake well.

For direct application:

Blend the oils with a carrier oil such as sweet almond or fractionated coconut oil. You will need 1 tablespoon of oil to the essential oils you use. You can also blend these oils with your favorite lotion before applying directly to the affected area.

Repeat as needed.

For a diffuser:

Instead of mixing your oils then blending them with a carrier oil, you are going to mix them then transfer them into your diffuser with some water. Turn on your diffuser and allow the rich scent to fill your home from morning until night.

Choose a diffuser that turns off automatically.

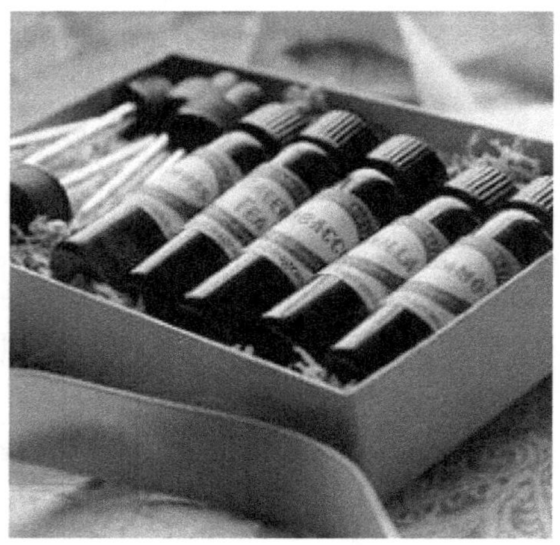

Forever Young

What you will need:

10 drops ylang ylang

11 drops vetiver oil

Directions:

In a small jar, combine all oils and shake well.

For direct application:

Blend the oils with a carrier oil such as sweet almond or fractionated coconut oil. You will need 1 tablespoon of oil to the essential oils you use. You can also blend these oils with your favorite lotion before applying directly to the affected area.

Repeat as needed.

For a diffuser:

Instead of mixing your oils then blending them with a carrier oil, you are going to mix them then transfer them into your diffuser with some water. Turn on your diffuser and allow the rich scent to fill your home from morning until night.

Choose a diffuser that turns off automatically.

Headache Healer
What you will need:

18 drops myrrh oil

15 drops bergamot

Directions:

In a small jar, combine all oils and shake well.

For direct application:

Blend the oils with a carrier oil such as sweet almond or fractionated coconut oil. You will need 1 tablespoon of oil to the essential oils you use. You can also blend these oils with your favorite lotion before applying directly to the affected area.

Repeat as needed.

For a diffuser:

Instead of mixing your oils then blending them with a carrier oil, you are going to mix them then transfer them into your diffuser with some water. Turn on your diffuser and allow the rich scent to fill your home from morning until night.

Choose a diffuser that turns off automatically.

Joint Juice
What you will need:

12 drops myrrh oil

12 drops lavender oil

Directions:

In a small jar, combine all oils and shake well.

For direct application:

Blend the oils with a carrier oil such as sweet almond or fractionated coconut oil. You will need 1 tablespoon of oil to the essential oils you use. You can also blend these oils with your favorite lotion before applying directly to the affected area.

Repeat as needed.

For a diffuser:

Instead of mixing your oils then blending them with a carrier oil, you are going to mix them then transfer them into your diffuser with some water. Turn on your diffuser and allow the rich scent to fill your home from morning until night.

Choose a diffuser that turns off automatically.

Elegant Goddess
What you will need:

9 drops goldenseal oil

11 drops lemongrass oil

Directions:

In a small jar, combine all oils and shake well.

For direct application:

Blend the oils with a carrier oil such as sweet almond or fractionated coconut oil. You will need 1 tablespoon of oil to the essential oils you use. You can also blend these oils with your favorite lotion before applying directly to the affected area.

Repeat as needed.

For a diffuser:

Instead of mixing your oils then blending them with a carrier oil, you are going to mix them then transfer them into your diffuser with some water. Turn on your diffuser and allow the rich scent to fill your home from morning until night.

Choose a diffuser that turns off automatically.

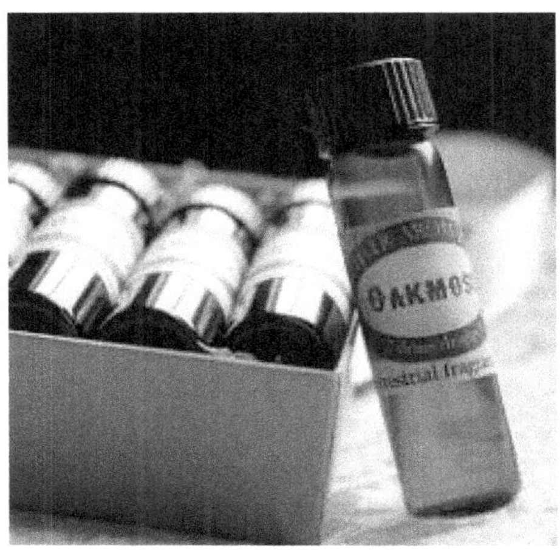

Wrinkle Eraser
What you will need:

15 drops myrrh oil

12 drops grapefruit oil

Directions:

In a small jar, combine all oils and shake well.

For direct application:

Blend the oils with a carrier oil such as sweet almond or fractionated coconut oil. You will need 1 tablespoon of oil to the essential oils you use. You can also blend these oils with your favorite lotion before applying directly to the affected area.

Repeat as needed.

For a diffuser:

Instead of mixing your oils then blending them with a carrier oil, you are going to mix them then transfer them into your diffuser with some water. Turn on your diffuser and allow the rich scent to fill your home from morning until night.

Choose a diffuser that turns off automatically.

Arthritis Ambush

What you will need:

19 drops peppermint oil

15 drops myrrh oil

Directions:

In a small jar, combine all oils and shake well.

For direct application:

Blend the oils with a carrier oil such as sweet almond or fractionated coconut oil. You will need 1 tablespoon of oil to the essential oils you use. You can also blend these oils with your favorite lotion before applying directly to the affected area.

Repeat as needed.

For a diffuser:

Instead of mixing your oils then blending them with a carrier oil, you are going to mix them then transfer them into your diffuser with some water. Turn on your diffuser and allow the rich scent to fill your home from morning until night.

Choose a diffuser that turns off automatically.

Spring Day
What you will need:

10 drops lavender oil

12 drops rose oil

Directions:

In a small jar, combine all oils and shake well.

For direct application:

Blend the oils with a carrier oil such as sweet almond or fractionated coconut oil. You will need 1 tablespoon of oil to the essential oils you use. You can also blend these oils with your favorite lotion before applying directly to the affected area.

Repeat as needed.

For a diffuser:

Instead of mixing your oils then blending them with a carrier oil, you are going to mix them then transfer them into your diffuser with some water. Turn on your diffuser and allow the rich scent to fill your home from morning until night.

Choose a diffuser that turns off automatically.

Good Night's Sleep

What you will need:

10 drops lavender oil

12 drops chamomile oil

Directions:

In a small jar, combine all oils and shake well.

For direct application:

Blend the oils with a carrier oil such as sweet almond or fractionated coconut oil. You will need 1 tablespoon of oil to the essential oils you use. You can also blend these oils with your favorite lotion before applying directly to the affected area.

Repeat as needed.

For a diffuser:

Instead of mixing your oils then blending them with a carrier oil, you are going to mix them then transfer them into your diffuser with some water. Turn on your diffuser and allow the rich scent to fill your home from morning until night.

Choose a diffuser that turns off automatically.

Beauty

What you will need:

11 drops sandalwood oil

12 drops rosewood oil

Directions:

In a small jar, combine all oils and shake well.

For direct application:

Blend the oils with a carrier oil such as sweet almond or fractionated coconut oil. You will need 1 tablespoon of oil to the essential oils you use. You can also blend these oils with your favorite lotion before applying directly to the affected area.

Repeat as needed.

For a diffuser:

Instead of mixing your oils then blending them with a carrier oil, you are going to mix them then transfer them into your diffuser with some water. Turn on your diffuser and allow the rich scent to fill your home from morning until night.

Choose a diffuser that turns off automatically.

The Nightingale

What you will need:

12 drops geranium oil

10 drops cedar oil

Directions:

In a small jar, combine all oils and shake well.

For direct application:

Blend the oils with a carrier oil such as sweet almond or fractionated coconut oil. You will need 1 tablespoon of oil to the essential oils you use. You can also blend these oils with your favorite lotion before applying directly to the affected area.

Repeat as needed.

For a diffuser:

Instead of mixing your oils then blending them with a carrier oil, you are going to mix them then transfer them into your diffuser with some water. Turn on your diffuser and allow the rich scent to fill your home from morning until night.

Choose a diffuser that turns off automatically.

Meadow Blooms

What you will need:

10 drops roman chamomile oil

10 drops chamomile oil

Directions:

In a small jar, combine all oils and shake well.

For direct application:

Blend the oils with a carrier oil such as sweet almond or fractionated coconut oil. You will need 1 tablespoon of oil to the essential oils you use. You can also blend these oils with your favorite lotion before applying directly to the affected area.

Repeat as needed.

For a diffuser:

Instead of mixing your oils then blending them with a carrier oil, you are going to mix them then transfer them into your diffuser with some water. Turn on your diffuser and allow the rich scent to fill your home from morning until night.

Choose a diffuser that turns off automatically.

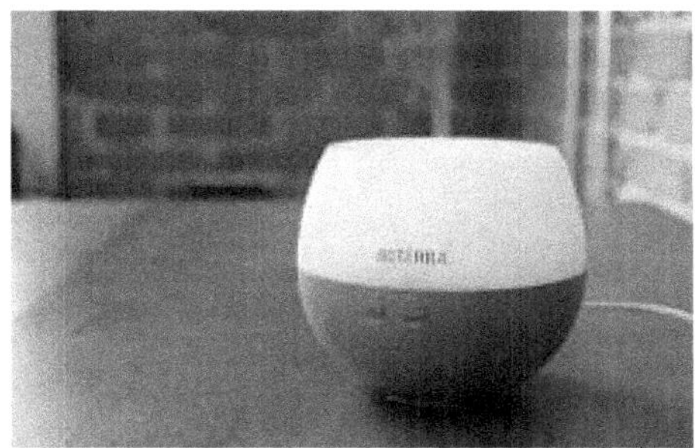

Happiness

What you will need:

12 drops vetiver oil

11 drops winter green oil

Directions:

In a small jar, combine all oils and shake well.

For direct application:

Blend the oils with a carrier oil such as sweet almond or fractionated coconut oil. You will need 1 tablespoon of oil to the essential oils you use. You can also blend these oils with your favorite lotion before applying directly to the affected area.

Repeat as needed.

For a diffuser:

Instead of mixing your oils then blending them with a carrier oil, you are going to mix them then transfer them into your diffuser with some water. Turn on your diffuser and allow the rich scent to fill your home from morning until night.

Choose a diffuser that turns off automatically.

Earth Days

What you will need:

10 drops sandalwood oil

11 drops pine oil

Directions:

In a small jar, combine all oils and shake well.

For direct application:

Blend the oils with a carrier oil such as sweet almond or fractionated coconut oil. You will need 1 tablespoon of oil to the essential oils you use. You can also blend these oils with your favorite lotion before applying directly to the affected area.

Repeat as needed.

For a diffuser:

Instead of mixing your oils then blending them with a carrier oil, you are going to mix them then transfer them into your diffuser with some water. Turn on your diffuser and allow the rich scent to fill your home from morning until night.

Choose a diffuser that turns off automatically.

Heavenly Sunset

What you will need:

10 drops lemon oil

11 drops blood orange oil

Directions:

In a small jar, combine all oils and shake well.

For direct application:

Blend the oils with a carrier oil such as sweet almond or fractionated coconut oil. You will need 1 tablespoon of oil to the essential oils you use. You can also blend these oils with your favorite lotion before applying directly to the affected area.

Repeat as needed.

For a diffuser:

Instead of mixing your oils then blending them with a carrier oil, you are going to mix them then transfer them into your diffuser with some water. Turn on your diffuser and allow the rich scent to fill your home from morning until night.

Choose a diffuser that turns off automatically.

Sunshine on My Shoulders

What you will need:

10 drops vanilla oil

11 drops rose oil

Directions:

In a small jar, combine all oils and shake well.

For direct application:

Blend the oils with a carrier oil such as sweet almond or fractionated coconut oil. You will need 1 tablespoon of oil to the essential oils you use. You can also blend these oils with your favorite lotion before applying directly to the affected area.

Repeat as needed.

For a diffuser:

Instead of mixing your oils then blending them with a carrier oil, you are going to mix them then transfer them into your diffuser with some water. Turn on your diffuser and allow the rich scent to fill your home from morning until night.

Choose a diffuser that turns off automatically.

Move Freely
What you will need:

12 drops myrrh oil

12 drops vanilla oil

Directions:

In a small jar, combine all oils and shake well.

For direct application:

Blend the oils with a carrier oil such as sweet almond or fractionated coconut oil. You will need 1 tablespoon of oil to the essential oils you use. You can also blend these oils with your favorite lotion before applying directly to the affected area.

Repeat as needed.

For a diffuser:

Instead of mixing your oils then blending them with a carrier oil, you are going to mix them then transfer them into your diffuser with some water. Turn on your diffuser and allow the rich scent to fill your home from morning until night.

Choose a diffuser that turns off automatically.

The Up Side
What you will need:

11 drops lemongrass oil

10 drops white fir needle oil

Directions:

In a small jar, combine all oils and shake well.

For direct application:

Blend the oils with a carrier oil such as sweet almond or fractionated coconut oil. You will need 1 tablespoon of oil to the essential oils you use. You can also blend these oils with your favorite lotion before applying directly to the affected area.

Repeat as needed.

For a diffuser:

Instead of mixing your oils then blending them with a carrier oil, you are going to mix them then transfer them into your diffuser with some water. Turn on your diffuser and allow the rich scent to fill your home from morning until night.

Choose a diffuser that turns off automatically.

Grace

What you will need:

10 drops cardamom oil

10 drops vetiver oil

Directions:

In a small jar, combine all oils and shake well.

For direct application:

Blend the oils with a carrier oil such as sweet almond or fractionated coconut oil. You will need 1 tablespoon of oil to the essential oils you use. You can also blend these oils with your favorite lotion before applying directly to the affected area.

Repeat as needed.

For a diffuser:

Instead of mixing your oils then blending them with a carrier oil, you are going to mix them then transfer them into your diffuser with some water. Turn on your diffuser and allow the rich scent to fill your home from morning until night.

Choose a diffuser that turns off automatically.

Blessed Movement

What you will need:

10 drops peppermint oil

8 drops spearmint oil

Directions:

In a small jar, combine all oils and shake well.

For direct application:

Blend the oils with a carrier oil such as sweet almond or fractionated coconut oil. You will need 1 tablespoon of oil to the essential oils you use. You can also blend these oils with your favorite lotion before applying directly to the affected area.

Repeat as needed.

For a diffuser:

Instead of mixing your oils then blending them with a carrier oil, you are going to mix them then transfer them into your diffuser with some water. Turn on your diffuser and allow the rich scent to fill your home from morning until night.

Choose a diffuser that turns off automatically.

Get Up and Go
What you will need:

15 drops eucalyptus oil

10 drops grapefruit oil

Directions:

In a small jar, combine all oils and shake well.

For direct application:

Blend the oils with a carrier oil such as sweet almond or fractionated coconut oil. You will need 1 tablespoon of oil to the essential oils you use. You can also blend these oils with your favorite lotion before applying directly to the affected area.

Repeat as needed.

For a diffuser:

Instead of mixing your oils then blending them with a carrier oil, you are going to mix them then transfer them into your diffuser with some water. Turn on your diffuser and allow the rich scent to fill your home from morning until night.

Choose a diffuser that turns off automatically.

Tummy Trouble
What you will need:

10 drops peppermint oil

8 drops tea tree oil

Directions:

In a small jar, combine all oils and shake well.

For direct application:

Blend the oils with a carrier oil such as sweet almond or fractionated coconut oil. You will need 1 tablespoon of oil to the essential oils you use. You can also blend these oils with your favorite lotion before applying directly to the affected area.

Repeat as needed.

For a diffuser:

Instead of mixing your oils then blending them with a carrier oil, you are going to mix them then transfer them into your diffuser with some water. Turn on your diffuser and allow the rich scent to fill your home from morning until night.

Choose a diffuser that turns off automatically.

Green Thumb
What you will need:

10 drops patchouli oil

10 drops cedar oil

Directions:

In a small jar, combine all oils and shake well.

For direct application:

Blend the oils with a carrier oil such as sweet almond or fractionated coconut oil. You will need 1 tablespoon of oil to the essential oils you use. You can also blend these oils with your favorite lotion before applying directly to the affected area.

Repeat as needed.

For a diffuser:

Instead of mixing your oils then blending them with a carrier oil, you are going to mix them then transfer them into your diffuser with some water. Turn on your diffuser and allow the rich scent to fill your home from morning until night.

Choose a diffuser that turns off automatically.

Smiley Days

What you will need:

10 drops jasmine oil

10 drops juniper berry oil

Directions:

In a small jar, combine all oils and shake well.

For direct application:

Blend the oils with a carrier oil such as sweet almond or fractionated coconut oil. You will need 1 tablespoon of oil to the essential oils you use. You can also blend these oils with your favorite lotion before applying directly to the affected area.

Repeat as needed.

For a diffuser:

Instead of mixing your oils then blending them with a carrier oil, you are going to mix them then transfer them into your diffuser with some water. Turn on your diffuser and allow the rich scent to fill your home from morning until night.

Choose a diffuser that turns off automatically.

Year Round Wonder

What you will need:

19 drops bergamot oil

10 drops patchouli oil

Directions:

In a small jar, combine all oils and shake well.

For direct application:

Blend the oils with a carrier oil such as sweet almond or fractionated coconut oil. You will need 1 tablespoon of oil to the essential oils you use. You can also blend these oils with your favorite lotion before applying directly to the affected area.

Repeat as needed.

For a diffuser:

Instead of mixing your oils then blending them with a carrier oil, you are going to mix them then transfer them into your diffuser with some water. Turn on your diffuser and allow the rich scent to fill your home from morning until night.

Choose a diffuser that turns off automatically.

The Glow

What you will need:

9 drops goldenseal

8 drops ylang ylang

Directions:

In a small jar, combine all oils and shake well.

For direct application:

Blend the oils with a carrier oil such as sweet almond or fractionated coconut oil. You will need 1 tablespoon of oil to the essential oils you use. You can also blend these oils with your favorite lotion before applying directly to the affected area.

Repeat as needed.

For a diffuser:

Instead of mixing your oils then blending them with a carrier oil, you are going to mix them then transfer them into your diffuser with some water. Turn on your diffuser and allow the rich scent to fill your home from morning until night.

Choose a diffuser that turns off automatically.

Morning Mist
What you will need:

10 drops lavender oil

10 drops eucalyptus oil

Directions:

In a small jar, combine all oils and shake well.

For direct application:

Blend the oils with a carrier oil such as sweet almond or fractionated coconut oil. You will need 1 tablespoon of oil to the essential oils you use. You can also blend these oils with your favorite lotion before applying directly to the affected area.

Repeat as needed.

For a diffuser:

Instead of mixing your oils then blending them with a carrier oil, you are going to mix them then transfer them into your diffuser with some water. Turn on your diffuser and allow the rich scent to fill your home from morning until night.

Choose a diffuser that turns off automatically.

Magic Blend

What you will need:

10 drops clove oil

17 drops ginger oil

Directions:

In a small jar, combine all oils and shake well.

For direct application:

Blend the oils with a carrier oil such as sweet almond or fractionated coconut oil. You will need 1 tablespoon of oil to the essential oils you use. You can also blend these oils with your favorite lotion before applying directly to the affected area.

Repeat as needed.

For a diffuser:

Instead of mixing your oils then blending them with a carrier oil, you are going to mix them then transfer them into your diffuser with some water. Turn on your diffuser and allow the rich scent to fill your home from morning until night.

Choose a diffuser that turns off automatically.

Ooh La La
What you will need:

10 drops sunflower essential oil

8 drops vanilla oil

Directions:

In a small jar, combine all oils and shake well.

For direct application:

Blend the oils with a carrier oil such as sweet almond or fractionated coconut oil. You will need 1 tablespoon of oil to the essential oils you use. You can also blend these oils with your favorite lotion before applying directly to the affected area.

Repeat as needed.

For a diffuser:

Instead of mixing your oils then blending them with a carrier oil, you are going to mix them then transfer them into your diffuser with some water. Turn on your diffuser and allow the rich scent to fill your home from morning until night.

Choose a diffuser that turns off automatically.

Your Favorite Blend
What you will need:

10 drops spearmint oil

10 drops winter green oil

Directions:

In a small jar, combine all oils and shake well.

For direct application:

Blend the oils with a carrier oil such as sweet almond or fractionated coconut oil. You will need 1 tablespoon of oil to the essential oils you use. You can also blend these oils with your favorite lotion before applying directly to the affected area.

Repeat as needed.

For a diffuser:

Instead of mixing your oils then blending them with a carrier oil, you are going to mix them then transfer them into your diffuser with some water. Turn on your diffuser and allow the rich scent to fill your home from morning until night.

Choose a diffuser that turns off automatically.

Better than the Best
What you will need:

7 drops pine oil

8 drops sandalwood oil

Directions:

In a small jar, combine all oils and shake well.

For direct application:

Blend the oils with a carrier oil such as sweet almond or fractionated coconut oil. You will need 1 tablespoon of oil to the essential oils you use. You can also blend these oils with your favorite lotion before applying directly to the affected area.

Repeat as needed.

For a diffuser:

Instead of mixing your oils then blending them with a carrier oil, you are going to mix them then transfer them into your diffuser with some water. Turn on your diffuser and allow the rich scent to fill your home from morning until night.

Choose a diffuser that turns off automatically.

Spring Chicken
What you will need:

10 drops orange oil

8 drops blood orange oil

Directions:

In a small jar, combine all oils and shake well.

For direct application:

Blend the oils with a carrier oil such as sweet almond or fractionated coconut oil. You will need 1 tablespoon of oil to the essential oils you use. You can also blend these oils with your favorite lotion before applying directly to the affected area.

Repeat as needed.

For a diffuser:

Instead of mixing your oils then blending them with a carrier oil, you are going to mix them then transfer them into your diffuser with some water. Turn on your diffuser and allow the rich scent to fill your home from morning until night.

Choose a diffuser that turns off automatically.

Early Bird Special
What you will need:

10 drops rose oil

9 drops basil oil

Directions:

In a small jar, combine all oils and shake well.

For direct application:

Blend the oils with a carrier oil such as sweet almond or fractionated coconut oil. You will need 1 tablespoon of oil to the essential oils you use. You can also blend these oils with your favorite lotion before applying directly to the affected area.

Repeat as needed.

For a diffuser:

Instead of mixing your oils then blending them with a carrier oil, you are going to mix them then transfer them into your diffuser with some water. Turn on your diffuser and allow the rich scent to fill your home from morning until night.

Choose a diffuser that turns off automatically.

Magic Spritz
What you will need:

10 drops geranium oil

5 drops vetiver oil

Directions:

In a small jar, combine all oils and shake well.

For direct application:

Blend the oils with a carrier oil such as sweet almond or fractionated coconut oil. You will need 1 tablespoon of oil to the essential oils you use. You can also blend these oils with your favorite lotion before applying directly to the affected area.

Repeat as needed.

For a diffuser:

Instead of mixing your oils then blending them with a carrier oil, you are going to mix them then transfer them into your diffuser with some water. Turn on your diffuser and allow the rich scent to fill your home from morning until night.

Choose a diffuser that turns off automatically.

Make a Splash
What you will need:

10 drops grapefruit oil

7 drops rose oil

3 drops lemon oil

Directions:

In a small jar, combine all oils and shake well.

For direct application:

Blend the oils with a carrier oil such as sweet almond or fractionated coconut oil. You will need 1 tablespoon of oil to the essential oils you use. You can also blend these oils with your favorite lotion before applying directly to the affected area.

Repeat as needed.

For a diffuser:

Instead of mixing your oils then blending them with a carrier oil, you are going to mix them then transfer them into your diffuser with some water. Turn on your diffuser and allow the rich scent to fill your home from morning until night.

Choose a diffuser that turns off automatically.

Conclusion

There you have it, everything you need to know to make your own essential oil blends, and to enjoy a life of greater movement, fewer wrinkles, and more comfort. You know the aches and pains that come with aging, but you don't have to turn to the pills that are offered in many of the stores.

With the essential oil blends, you can alleviate any of those aches and pains easily, knowing that you are going to be able to feel younger, look younger, and enjoy your life as you always have.

Mix the blends and use them in your diffuser, or apply them to your skin directly – either way, you are going to get the amazing benefits you deserve.

Happy blending!

FREE Bonus Reminder

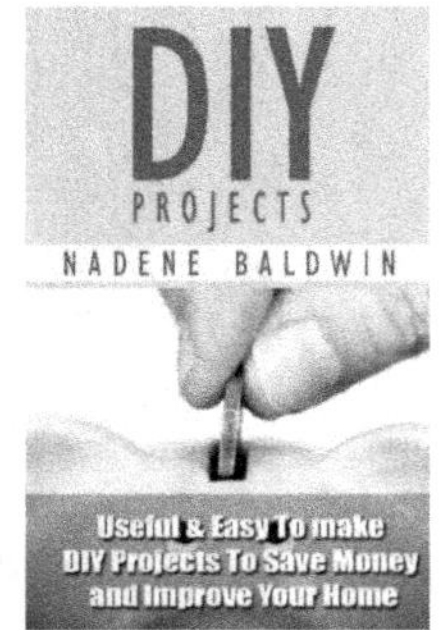

If you have not grabbed it yet, please go ahead and download your special bonus report *"DIY Projects. 13 Useful & Easy To Make DIY Projects To Save Money & Improve Your Home!"*
Simply Click the Button Below

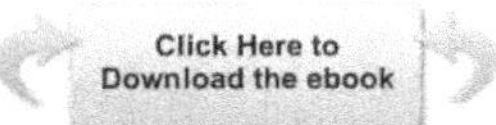

OR **Go to This Page**
http://diyhomecraft.com/free

BONUS #2: More Free & Discounted Books or Products

Do you want to receive more Free/Discounted Books or Products?
We have a mailing list where we send out our new Books or Products when they go free or with a discount on Amazon. Click on the link below to sign up for Free & Discount Book & Product Promotions.
=> Sign Up for Free & Discount Book & Product Promotions <=

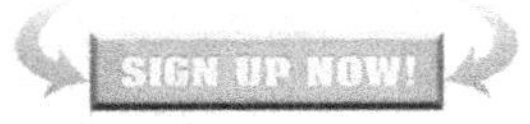

OR Go to this URL
http://bit.ly/1WBb1Ek

9 781978 342927